THE WHAT TO EXPECT WHEN YOU'RE EXPECTING

PREGNANCY ORGANIZER

By Arlene Eisenberg,
Heidi E. Murkoff, and
Sandee E. Hathaway, B.S.N.

WORKMAN PUBLISHING, NEW YORK

Published simultaneously in Canada by Thomas Allen & Son Limited.

Cover and book design: Janet Vicario
Cover illustration: Judith Cheng

Workman Publishing Company, Inc.
708 Broadway
New York, NY 10003

Manufactured in the United States of America
First printing June 1995
10 9 8 7 6 5 4 3 2

The Pregnancy Organizer

To record every highlight of your pregnancy, from your first reactions through your last contractions; to keep track of every detail, from your health to your finances, from your daily diet to your weekly weight gain to your monthly checkups, from your insurance paperwork to your childbirth class homework; to plan ahead and prepare for baby's arrival, from layette shopping to birth announcing—*The Pregnancy Organizer* can help you take charge of one of the happiest, and most complicated, times of your life.

Prenatal Care

1

Prenatal Care

Why should you record every little detail—physical, emotional, medical, financial—of your pregnancy? So you'll never have to ask yourself, "Why didn't I record...?" So when you choose a different obstetrician or a midwife for your next pregnancy, you'll be able to recall the medical particulars of your first. So when you want to compare notes (when did morning sickness stop and indigestion take over?) with your newly pregnant sister-in-law, you'll have notes to compare. So when you find yourself in a postpartum dispute with the insurance company, you'll have records to show to support your claim. So when you simply want to reminisce, you'll be able to conjure up more than just a nine-month blur.

Of course, you can't record what you don't know. Don't hesitate to ask your practitioner for the results of any test—from monthly blood pressure readings to one-time blood or other diagnostic tests. Don't hesitate, either, to tap your practitioner as a resource at, or between, office visits. Jot down your questions as they come up (you're sure to forget them otherwise) and your practitioner's answers as you get them (or you'll forget those, too). Also record all medications you take (and take only those prescribed by your practitioner).

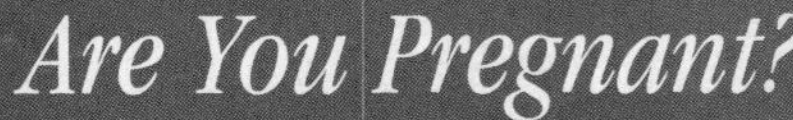

Are You Pregnant?

First Signs of Pregnancy

Use this page to record the date each sign was first noticed.

Date of your last menstrual period April 27, 1998

Menstrual period was due May 26, 1998

Morning (or any-time-of-day) sickness morning/Night - after not eating for long periods

Breast changes:

x enlargement

x tingling, tenderness

darkening of the areola (area around your nipple)

prominence of tiny glands around nipple

appearance of blue and pink lines (blood vessels) under skin

Frequent urination yes - especially in the middle of the night

Food cravings

Aversions Strong smells upset my stomach

Other

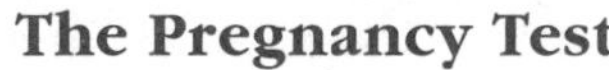

Are You Pregnant?

The Pregnancy Test

Date taken ______ Where Home

Type of test Home Pregnancy Test

Results Positive

Date results received ______ From whom ______

Repeat Pregnancy Test

Date taken ______ Where Home

Type of test Home Pregnancy test

Results Positive

Date results received ______ From whom ______

Repeat Pregnancy Test

Date taken ______ Where ______

Type of test ______

Results ______

Date results received ______ From whom ______

Repeat Pregnancy Test

Date taken ______ Where ______

Type of test ______

Results ______

Date results received ______ From whom ______

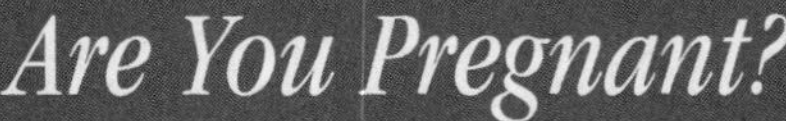

Are You Pregnant?

Repeat Pregnancy Test

Date taken Where

Type of test

Results

Date results received From whom

Repeat Pregnancy Test

Date taken Where

Type of test

Results

Date results received From whom

Physical Exam to Verify Pregnancy

Practitioner Date

Findings

Estimated due date

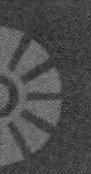

Congratulations!

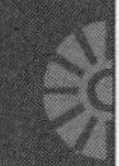

Your reaction

Your spouse/partner's reaction

Reactions of other children, if any

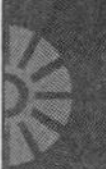

Congratulations!

Reactions of grandparents

Reactions of friends

How you celebrated

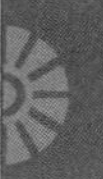

Your Practitioner

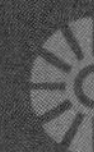

Name

Address

Phone

Associates, if any

Office hours

Call hours

Protocol to follow in emergencies (when to call, what to do if you can't reach your practitioner)

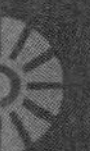

Personal Health History

Discuss the following with your practitioner at the first visit.

Your present health

Chronic conditions None

Medication taken regularly None

Other

Personal Health History

Your reproductive history

Fertility issues and treatment, if any

Number of previous pregnancies 1

Spontaneous miscarriage(s); dates and possible cause(s)

2nd trimester miscarriage - 3/94

cause - not know

Pregnancy termination(s); dates and complications, if any

Complications in previous pregnancies

Prior delivery complications

Type(s) of delivery

Personal Health History

Your lifestyle

Do you smoke? NO

Do you use alcohol or other drugs (be specific–and honest–as to type of drug, frequency, and amount)? alcohol - 1-2 drinks/mont

Do you exercise? If so, what type(s) of exercise, and how often?

Do you have a cat? no Does it spend time outdoors?

Do you take vitamins or any herbal preparations? If so what kinds? not regularly

Possible exposure to environmental hazards

At work –

At home –

Other concerns

I am very concerned about my weight -

High blood pressure

gestational Diabetes

miscarriage.

Personal & Family Health History

Condition	You	Baby's father	Baby's sibs	Parent's sibs*	Grand-parents*
Allergies					
Asthma					
Birth defects**					
Cancer					
Cystic fibrosis					
Diabetes					
Drug/alcohol abuse					
Heart problems					
Hypertension					
Hemophilia					
Down syndrome					
Mental retardation					
Muscular dystrophy					
PKU (phenylketonuria)					
Sickle-cell anemia					
Spina bifida					
Tay-Sachs disease					
Thalassemia					
Other**					
Other**					

*Indicate M for maternal siblings/grandparents, P for paternal siblings/grandparents.

**Other than those listed.

Your Baseline Medical Record

During your first prenatal exam, your practitioner will probably check most or all of the following. Use this space to record the results.

Weight __________

Blood pressure __________

Pulse __________

Breast exam __________

Pap smear __________

Blood type __________

Hemoglobin or hematocrit __________

Urinalysis: sugar __________

protein __________

bacteria __________

Rubella titer __________

Gonorrhea culture __________

VDRL (for syphilis) __________

Genital herpes __________

Chlamydia __________

Toxoplasmosis __________

HIV (human immunodeficiency virus) __________

Drug screen __________

Chronic illness(es) __________

Other __________

Father's blood type, if relevant __________

Practitioner's Recommendations

Jot down your practitioner's recommendations for dealing with the following during your pregnancy.

Prescription medications

Over-the-counter medications

Diet

Exercise

Lovemaking/orgasm

Work

Practitioner's Recommendations

Travel

Limitations on activities, if any

Steps to take concerning potential environmental hazards at home/at work

Symptoms warranting a call

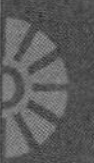

Prenatal Diagnosis

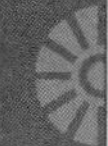

Maternal Serum Screenings

Maternal serum alpha-fetoprotein screening (MSAFP)

Date/Place

Practitioner

Results

Comments

Human chorionic gonadotrophin (hCG)

Date/Place

Practitioner

Results

Comments

Maternal serum unconjugated estriol

Date/Place

Practitioner

Results

Comments

Followup tests needed, if any

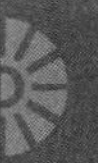

Prenatal Diagnosis

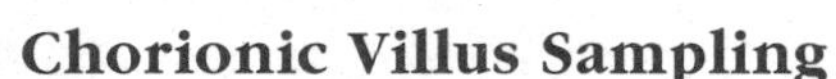

Chorionic Villus Sampling

Date/Place

Practitioner

Results

Comments

Amniocentesis

Date/Place

Practitioner

Results

Comments

Prenatal Diagnosis

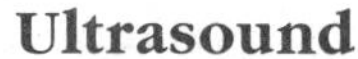

Ultrasound

Date/Place July 10, 1998 Rome Hospital

Practitioner

Results 10 wks 3 days old -
Heartbeat 163 beats/min

Rome was with me.

Comments The technician said the baby was moving all around - I heard the heartbeat - it was amazing

Ultrasound

Date/Place

Practitioner

Results

Comments

Ultrasound

Date/Place

Practitioner

Results

Comments

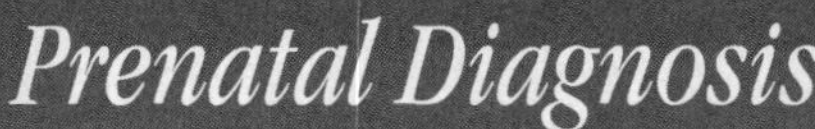

Prenatal Diagnosis

Toxoplasmosis

Date/Place

Practitioner/Technician

Results

Comments

Hepatitis B Screen

Date (usually late in second trimester) Place

Practitioner/Technician

Results

Comments

Group B Strep Swab

Date (at 26–28 weeks) Place

Practitioner/Technician

Results

Comments

Glucose Tolerance Test

Date (usually in fifth month) Place

Practitioner/Technician

Results

Comments

Other Tests

Date/Place

Practitioner/Technician

Results

Comments

Date/Place

Practitioner/Technician

Results

Comments

Notes

Practitioner's Visit Record

Practitioner seen

Date/Time

Weight

Blood Pressure Pulse

Urinalysis: sugar protein

Other tests

Height of fundus

Fetal heart rate (usually first detected between 10–18 weeks)

Comments

Practitioner's Instructions

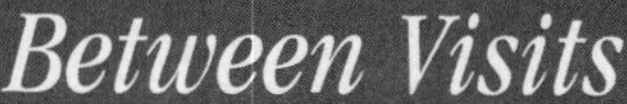

Between Visits

Calls Made to Practitioner

Date called

Reason

Instructions

Date called

Reason

Instructions

Date called

Reason

Instructions

Questions to Ask at the Next Visit

Practitioner's Visit Record

Practitioner seen

Date/Time

Weight

Blood Pressure | Pulse

Urinalysis: sugar | protein

Other tests

Height of fundus

Fetal heart rate (usually first detected between 10–18 weeks)

Comments

Practitioner's Instructions

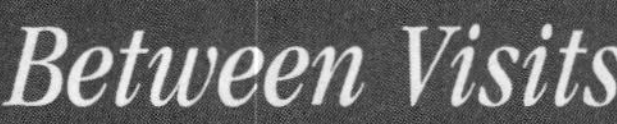

Between Visits

Calls Made to Practitioner

Date called

Reason

Instructions

Date called

Reason

Instructions

Date called

Reason

Instructions

Questions to Ask at the Next Visit

Practitioner's Visit Record

Practitioner seen

Date/Time

Weight

Blood Pressure Pulse

Urinalysis: sugar protein

Other tests

Height of fundus

Fetal heart rate (usually first detected between 10–18 weeks)

Comments

Practitioner's Instructions

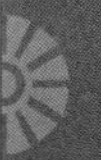

Between Visits

Calls Made to Practitioner

Date called

Reason

Instructions

Date called

Reason

Instructions

Date called

Reason

Instructions

Questions to Ask at the Next Visit

Practitioner's Visit Record

Practitioner seen

Date/Time

Weight

Blood Pressure Pulse

Urinalysis: sugar protein

Other tests

Height of fundus

Fetal heart rate (usually first detected between 10–18 weeks)

Comments

Practitioner's Instructions

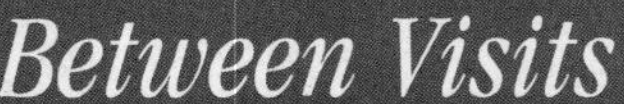

Between Visits

Calls Made to Practitioner

Date called

Reason

Instructions

Date called

Reason

Instructions

Date called

Reason

Instructions

Questions to Ask at the Next Visit

Practitioner's Visit Record

Practitioner seen

Date/Time

Weight

Blood Pressure Pulse

Urinalysis: sugar protein

Other tests

Height of fundus

Fetal heart rate (usually first detected between 10–18 weeks)

Comments

Practitioner's Instructions

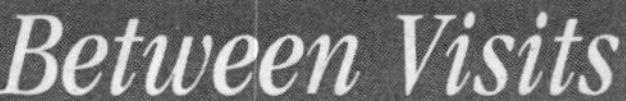

Between Visits

Calls Made to Practitioner

Date called

Reason

Instructions

Date called

Reason

Instructions

Date called

Reason

Instructions

Questions to Ask at the Next Visit

Practitioner's Visit Record

Practitioner seen

Date/Time

Weight

Blood Pressure | Pulse

Urinalysis: sugar | protein

Other tests

Height of fundus

Fetal heart rate

Comments

Practitioner's Instructions

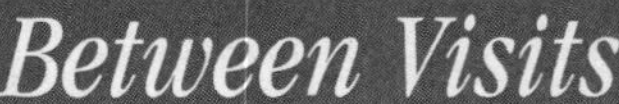

Between Visits

Calls Made to Practitioner

Date called

Reason

Instructions

Date called

Reason

Instructions

Date called

Reason

Instructions

Questions to Ask at the Next Visit

Practitioner's Visit Record

Practitioner seen

Date/Time

Weight

Blood Pressure Pulse

Urinalysis: sugar protein

Other tests

Height of fundus

Fetal heart rate

Comments

Practitioner's Instructions

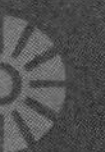

Calls Made to Practitioner

Date called

Reason

Instructions

Date called

Reason

Instructions

Date called

Reason

Instructions

Questions to Ask at the Next Visit

Practitioner's Visit Record

Practitioner seen

Date/Time

Weight

Blood Pressure | Pulse

Urinalysis: sugar | protein

Other tests

Height of fundus

Fetal heart rate

Comments

Practitioner's Instructions

Calls Made to Practitioner

Date called

Reason

Instructions

Date called

Reason

Instructions

Date called

Reason

Instructions

Questions to Ask at the Next Visit

Practitioner's Visit Record

Practitioner seen

Date/Time

Weight

Blood Pressure Pulse

Urinalysis: sugar protein

Other tests

Height of fundus

Fetal heart rate

Comments

Practitioner's Instructions

Between Visits

Calls Made to Practitioner

Date called

Reason

Instructions

Date called

Reason

Instructions

Date called

Reason

Instructions

Questions to Ask at the Next Visit

Practitioner's Visit Record

Practitioner seen

Date/Time

Weight

Blood Pressure Pulse

Urinalysis: sugar protein

Other tests

Height of fundus

Fetal heart rate

Comments

Practitioner's Instructions

Between Visits

Calls Made to Practitioner

Date called

Reason

Instructions

Date called

Reason

Instructions

Date called

Reason

Instructions

Questions to Ask at the Next Visit

Practitioner's Visit Record

Practitioner seen

Date/Time

Weight

Blood Pressure Pulse

Urinalysis: sugar protein

Other tests

Height of fundus

Fetal heart rate

Comments

Practitioner's Instructions

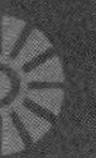

Between Visits

Calls Made to Practitioner

Date called

Reason

Instructions

Date called

Reason

Instructions

Date called

Reason

Instructions

Questions to Ask at the Next Visit

Practitioner's Visit Record

Practitioner seen

Date/Time

Weight

Blood Pressure Pulse

Urinalysis: sugar protein

Other tests

Height of fundus

Fetal heart rate

Comments

Practitioner's Instructions

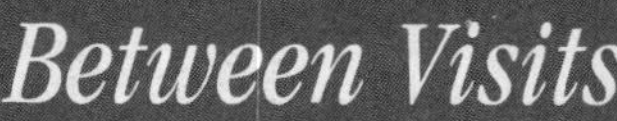

Between Visits

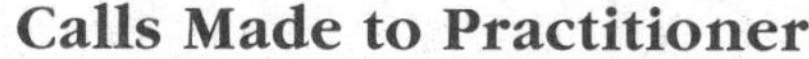

Calls Made to Practitioner

Date called

Reason

Instructions

Date called

Reason

Instructions

Date called

Reason

Instructions

Questions to Ask at the Next Visit

Practitioner's Visit Record

Practitioner seen

Date/Time

Weight

Blood Pressure | Pulse

Urinalysis: sugar | protein

Other tests

Height of fundus

Fetal heart rate

Comments

Practitioner's Instructions

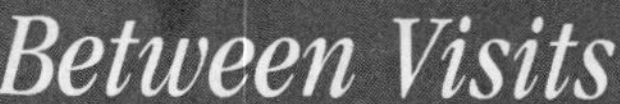

Between Visits

Calls Made to Practitioner

Date called

Reason

Instructions

Date called

Reason

Instructions

Date called

Reason

Instructions

Questions to Ask at the Next Visit

Practitioner's Visit Record

Practitioner seen

Date/Time

Weight

Blood Pressure Pulse

Urinalysis: sugar protein

Other tests

Height of fundus

Fetal heart rate

Comments

Practitioner's Instructions

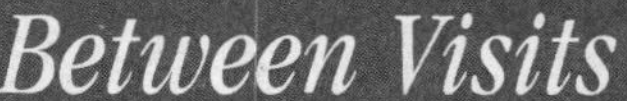

Between Visits

Calls Made to Practitioner

Date called

Reason

Instructions

Date called

Reason

Instructions

Date called

Reason

Instructions

Questions to Ask at the Next Visit

Prescribed Medications

Always be certain the prescribing physician knows you're pregnant.

Medication

Name Given for

Instructions

Prescription no.

Pharmacy name/address/phone

Date of original prescription Refills

Side effects/adverse reactions, if any

Discontinued on

Medication

Name Given for

Instructions

Prescription no.

Pharmacy name/address/phone

Date of original prescription Refills

Side effects/adverse reactions, if any

Discontinued on

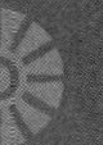

Prescribed Medications

Always be certain the prescribing physician knows you're pregnant.

Medication

Name Given for

Instructions

Prescription no.

Pharmacy name/address/phone

Date of original prescription Refills

Side effects/adverse reactions, if any

Discontinued on

Medication

Name Given for

Instructions

Prescription no.

Pharmacy name/address/phone

Date of original prescription Refills

Side effects/adverse reactions, if any

Discontinued on

Prescribed Medications

Always be certain the prescribing physician knows you're pregnant.

Medication

Name Given for

Instructions

Prescription no.

Pharmacy name/address/phone

Date of original prescription Refills

Side effects/adverse reactions, if any

Discontinued on

Medication

Name Given for

Instructions

Prescription no.

Pharmacy name/address/phone

Date of original prescription Refills

Side effects/adverse reactions, if any

Discontinued on

Over-the-Counter Medications

Don't take any medication without the approval of your practitioner.

Medication

Name Given for

Instructions

Pharmacy name/address/phone

Side effects/adverse reactions, if any

Discontinued on

Medication

Name Given for

Instructions

Pharmacy name/address/phone

Side effects/adverse reactions, if any

Discontinued on

Pregnancy-Related Medical Finances

Insurance company/HMO

Address

Phone

Policy holder's name and ID no.

Coverage

Contact person

Notes

Practitioner(s) providing prenatal care

Names

Address

Phone

Accepted method of payment

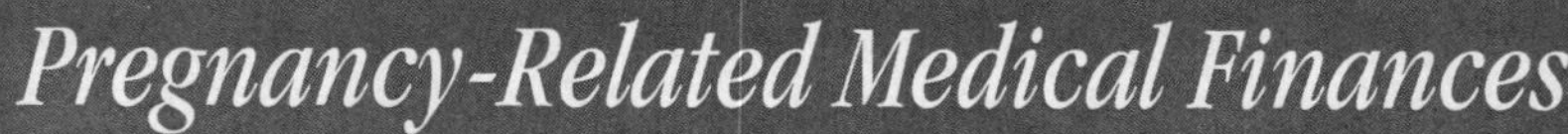

Pregnancy-Related Medical Finances

Use these pages to keep track of your pregnancy-related medical costs. As applicable, make note of payment schedules, bills received, bills submitted to your insurer, co-payments made, reimbursement received, and so on.

Your Practitioner

Other Pregnancy-Related Services

Service

Date provided

Provider

Address

Phone

Financial arrangement/fee

How paid Date paid

Notes

Service

Date provided

Provider

Address

Phone

Financial arrangement/fee

How paid Date paid

Notes

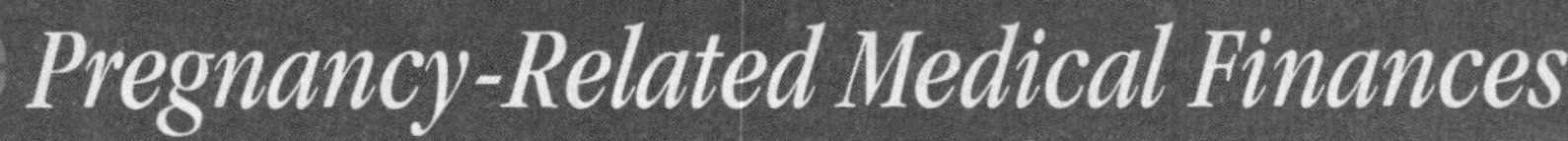

Other Pregnancy-Related Services

Service

Date provided

Provider

Address

Phone

Financial arrangement/fee

How paid Date paid

Notes

Service

Date provided

Provider

Address

Phone

Financial arrangement/fee

How paid Date paid

Notes

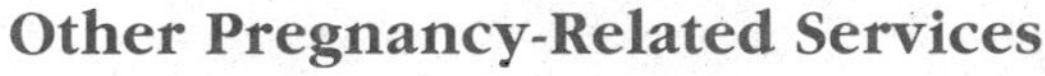

Other Pregnancy-Related Services

Service

Date provided

Provider

Address

Phone

Financial arrangement/fee

How paid Date paid

Notes

Service

Date provided

Provider

Address

Phone

Financial arrangement/fee

How paid Date paid

Notes

Other Pregnancy-Related Services

Service

Date provided

Provider

Address

Phone

Financial arrangement/fee

How paid   Date paid

Notes

Service

Date provided

Provider

Address

Phone

Financial arrangement/fee

How paid   Date paid

Notes

Other Pregnancy-Related Services

Service

Date provided

Provider

Address

Phone

Financial arrangement/fee

How paid Date paid

Notes

Service

Date provided

Provider

Address

Phone

Financial arrangement/fee

How paid Date paid

Notes

Other Pregnancy-Related Services

Service

Date provided

Provider

Address

Phone

Financial arrangement/fee

How paid Date paid

Notes

Service

Date provided

Provider

Address

Phone

Financial arrangement/fee

How paid Date paid

Notes

Notes

Notes

Your Pregnancy Journal

2

Your Pregnancy Journal

It may seem now as if everything that has happened or will happen to you during your pregnancy will be indelibly etched in your mind. But it won't be. And though there may be times when you'll want to forget these nine months, there will also be times when you'll want to look back and remember. To be sure your pregnancy experience *is* indelibly etched somewhere, use Your Weekly Pregnancy Diary pages to record your feelings and thoughts and those of your partner, along with milestones, special events, and so on.

Though details of your pregnancy may fade slowly over months or years, dietary memory may fade more quickly: You may not remember tomorrow what you ate today. Are you getting enough protein, calcium, and green leafy vegetables? Use the Daily Dozen Diary pages to keep track. You can check off each Daily Dozen requirement as it's filled or at the end of each day. By the time you're ready for bed, you'll know how close you've come to batting a Dozen. If you've come up short, a carefully chosen late night snack can help fill out your requirements.

The Pregnancy Wardrobe checklist can help with a less critical, but nevertheless important, pregnancy need: looking good.

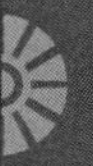

Your Weekly Pregnancy Diary

Record symptoms, feelings, milestones, and other special moments.

Week Number ___________ **Date**________________

Week Number ___________ **Date**________________

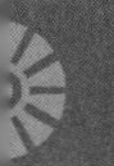

Your Weekly Pregnancy Diary

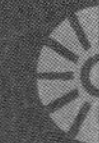

Record symptoms, feelings, milestones, and other special moments.

Week Number ___________ **Date**_______________

Week Number ___________ **Date**_______________

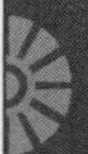

Your Weekly Pregnancy Diary

Record symptoms, feelings, milestones, and other special moments.

Week Number ____________ **Date**_________________

Week Number ____________ **Date**_________________

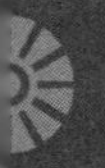

Your Weekly Pregnancy Diary

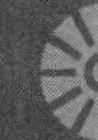

Record symptoms, feelings, milestones, and other special moments.

Week Number ___________ **Date**_______________

Week Number ___________ **Date**_______________

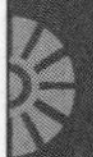

Your Weekly Pregnancy Diary

Record symptoms, feelings, milestones, and other special moments.

Week Number ____________ **Date**_________________

Week Number ____________ **Date**_________________

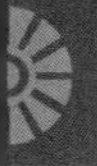

Your Weekly Pregnancy Diary

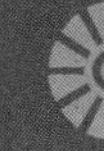

Record symptoms, feelings, milestones, and other special moments.

Week Number ____________ **Date**_________________

Week Number ____________ **Date**_________________

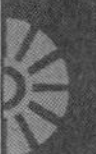

Your Weekly Pregnancy Diary

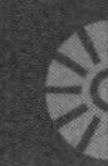

Record symptoms, feelings, milestones, and other special moments.

Week Number ___________ **Date**________________

Week Number ___________ **Date**________________

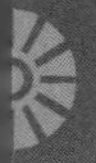

Your Weekly Pregnancy Diary

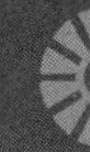

Record symptoms, feelings, milestones, and other special moments.

Week Number ____________ **Date**_________________

Week Number ____________ **Date**_________________

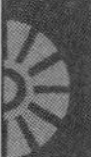

Your Weekly Pregnancy Diary

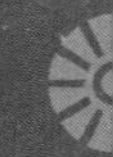

Record symptoms, feelings, milestones, and other special moments.

Week Number ____________ **Date**_________________

Week Number ____________ **Date**_________________

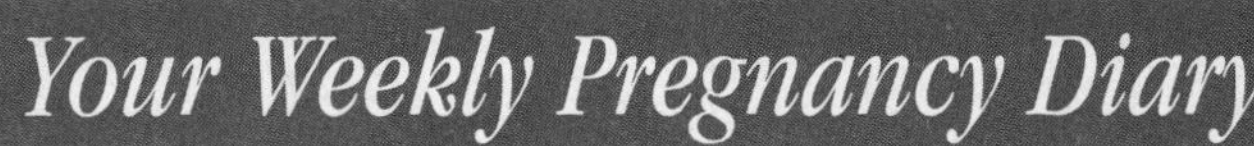

Your Weekly Pregnancy Diary

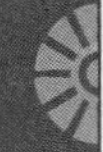

Record symptoms, feelings, milestones, and other special moments.

Week Number ____________ **Date**_________________

Week Number ____________ **Date**_________________

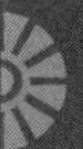

Your Weekly Pregnancy Diary

Record symptoms, feelings, milestones, and other special moments.

Week Number ___________ **Date**_______________

Week Number ___________ **Date**_______________

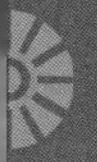

Your Weekly Pregnancy Diary

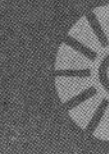

Record symptoms, feelings, milestones, and other special moments.

Week Number ____________ **Date**_________________

Week Number ____________ **Date**_________________

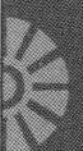

Your Weekly Pregnancy Diary

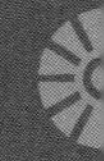

Record symptoms, feelings, milestones, and other special moments.

Week Number ____________ **Date**_________________

Week Number ____________ **Date**_________________

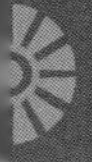

Your Weekly Pregnancy Diary

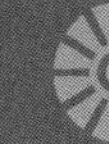

Record symptoms, feelings, milestones, and other special moments.

Week Number ____________ **Date**__________________

Week Number ____________ **Date**__________________

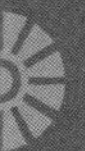

Your Weekly Pregnancy Diary

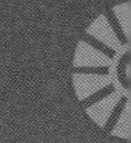

Record symptoms, feelings, milestones, and other special moments.

Week Number ____________ **Date**_________________

Week Number ____________ **Date**_________________

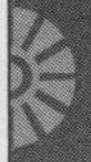

Your Weekly Pregnancy Diary

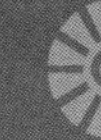

Record symptoms, feelings, milestones, and other special moments.

Week Number ___________ **Date**________________

Week Number ___________ **Date**________________

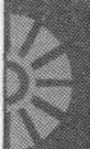

Your Weekly Pregnancy Diary

Record symptoms, feelings, milestones, and other special moments.

Week Number ___________ **Date**________________

Week Number ___________ **Date**________________

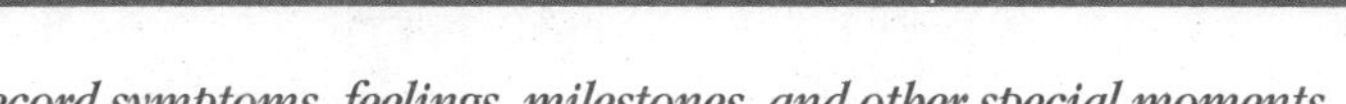

Your Weekly Pregnancy Diary

Record symptoms, feelings, milestones, and other special moments.

Week Number ____________ **Date** __________________

Week Number ____________ **Date** __________________

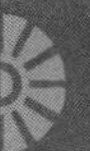

Your Weekly Pregnancy Diary

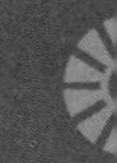

Record symptoms, feelings, milestones, and other special moments.

Week Number ____________ **Date**_________________

Week Number ____________ **Date**_________________

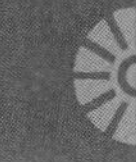

Your Weekly Pregnancy Diary

Record symptoms, feelings, milestones, and other special moments.

Week Number ___________ **Date**________________

Week Number ___________ **Date**________________

Your Weekly Pregnancy Diary

Record symptoms, feelings, milestones, and other special moments.

Week Number ___________ **Date**_______________

Week Number ___________ **Date**_______________

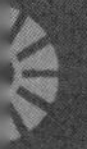

Fetal Movement Diary

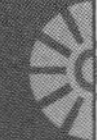

From the 28th week on, check for fetal movement twice daily, morning and evening. You should be able to detect 10 movements within a two hour period, though most of the time you will get to 10 in a much shorter time. Keep track below.

week	Sun. AM/PM		Mon. AM/PM		Tue. AM/PM		Wed. AM/PM		Thurs. AM/PM		Fri. AM/PM		Sat. AM/PM	
28														
29														
30														
31														
32														
33														
34														
35														
36														
37														
38														
39														
40														
41														
42														

The Daily Dozen

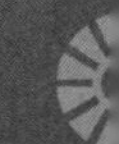

Each day you need:

1. Calories: Enough calories daily to keep you gaining at the rate of about a pound a month in the first trimester, ¾ to 1 pound per week in the fourth through eighth months, and 1 to 2 pounds (though you may not gain at all) in the ninth month, for a total of 25 to 35 pounds.

2. Protein Foods: Four 20- to 25-gram servings daily. One serving = 3½ ounces lean fish, meat, poultry, or hard cheese; 3 eggs or 1 whole egg plus 4 egg whites; ¾ cup low-fat cottage cheese; 3 cups skim milk; 5 to 6 ounces tofu; 1 cup beans with 1½ cups whole grains (rice, wheat, barley, oats, quinoa, bulgur, millet, etc.).

3. Vitamin C Foods: At least two 40- to 50-milligram servings daily. One serving = 6 ounces citrus juice; ½ grapefruit; 1 large orange; 1 medium mango; ¼ cantaloupe; 2 small tomatoes or 1¼ cups tomato juice; 1 cup vegetable juice; ½ medium green or ⅓ medium red bell pepper; ½ cup strawberries; ½ cup broccoli or ¾ cup cauliflower; 4 ounces raw spinach.

4. Calcium Foods: Four 300-milligram servings daily. One serving = 1 cup fresh or ½ cup evaporated or ⅓ cup nonfat dry skim milk; 1½ ounces hard cheese or 1¾ cups low-fat cottage cheese; 1 cup low-fat yogurt; 4 ounces canned salmon or sardines with bones; 1½ cups kale, mustard, or turnip greens; 2 cups broccoli; 2½ tablespoons blackstrap molasses; 1 cup calcium-added fruit juice. Ask your doctor to recommend a calcium supplement if you don't drink milk or eat other dairy products.

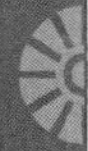

5. Green Leafy Vegetables and Yellow Fruits and Vegetables: At least three servings (each containing 1,500 to 2,000 IU vitamin A or the equivalent in beta-carotene) daily, preferably one green, one yellow, one raw. One serving = ¾ cup broccoli; ⅛ cantaloupe; ⅓ cup turnip greens, chard, or winter squash; 1 small carrot; ¼ cup kale or beet greens; 1 thick slice or 1 tablespoon yam or sweet potato; ¼ mango; 1 tablespoon puréed pumpkin; 8 large dark green lettuce leaves.

6. Other Fruits and Vegetables: At least two servings. One serving = 1 apple, pear, nectarine, or peach; 1 thick slice pineapple; 1 small potato; 6 asparagus spears; ⅔ cup Brussels sprouts or zucchini; ¾ cup green beans; ⅔ cup berries or cherries.

7. Whole Grains and Other Complex Carbohydrates: Five to 11 servings daily. One serving = 1 portion whole-grain bread, roll, muffin, pita, or bagel; 1 portion high-protein or whole-grain pasta, cooked brown rice, kasha, bulgur, millet, or other grain; 2 tablespoons wheat germ; 1 serving hot or cold whole-grain cereal.

8. Iron-Rich Foods: Some needed daily. Iron is found in liver and other organ meats (eat these rarely); clams and oysters (cooked only); soybeans and soy products; and blackstrap molasses. It is found in smaller quantities in beef; spinach, collards, kale, and turnip greens; legumes (dried peas and beans); spirulina (seaweed); dried figs, apricots, raisins, and other dried fruits. An iron supplement may be prescribed for you, especially if you're a vegetarian or you're anemic.

9. Fat: Get 30% of your calories from fat. That's about four 14- to 17-gram servings daily if your ideal prepregnancy weight was about 125 pounds and you're moderately active. You'll need fewer servings if you're inactive and/or weigh less (for example, 2½ servings for the inactive 100-pounder). You'll need more if you're very active and/or weigh more (about 7½ servings for a very active 150-pounder). One serving = 2 ounces Swiss, Cheddar, provolone, or mozzarella cheese; 3 ounces low-fat cheese; 1 tablespoon oil, butter, or mayonnaise; 2 tablespoons heavy cream or cream cheese; 1 cup ice cream; 2 whole eggs or yolks; 3 tablespoons nuts; ½ small avocado; 12 ounces tofu; 6 ounces tuna in oil; 7 ounces of dark-meat poultry (without skin); 3 to 6 ounces lean beef, veal, or pork; 8 ounces salmon. Though cholesterol is rarely a problem during pregnancy, you should still vary your fat sources and get more polyunsaturated and monosaturated fats (from olive and canola oils, for example) than saturated fats (such as butter or hydrogenated shortening).

10. Salt: Some sodium is needed daily, so salt your foods to taste in cooking and at the table. However, you should avoid overly salty foods (potato chips and pickles, for example); too much salt is not good for anyone.

11. Fluids: At least eight to ten 8-ounce glasses of fluid (water, juice, soup, or milk—not caffeinated tea or coffee) daily.

12. Nutritional Supplements: A pregnancy supplement daily (be sure it contains B_{12}, folic acid, zinc, and magnesium) is nutrition insurance. But it is not a substitute for eating the right foods.

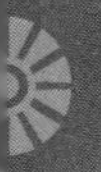

Your Daily Dozen Diary

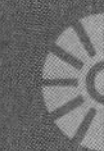

Check off each Daily Dozen serving daily. The number of servings you need per day appears in parentheses.

Month ___________ **Week** _________

	S	M	T	W	TH	F	S
Daily weight (optional)							
Protein foods (4)							
Vitamin C foods (2)							
Calcium foods (4)							
Green leafy/Yellows (3 or more)							
Other fruits & vegetables (2 or more)							
Grains/Carbs. (5 or more)							
Iron-rich foods (some daily)							
Fat (2½-7½)							
Salt							
Fluids (8-10)							
Nutritional supplement							

Month ___________ **Week** _________

	S	M	T	W	TH	F	S
Daily weight (optional)							
Protein foods (4)							
Vitamin C foods (2)							
Calcium foods (4)							
Green leafy/Yellows (3 or more)							
Other fruits & vegetables (2 or more)							
Grains/Carbs. (5 or more)							
Iron-rich foods (some daily)							
Fat (2½-7½)							
Salt							
Fluids (8-10)							
Nutritional supplement							

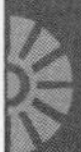

Your Daily Dozen Diary

Check off each Daily Dozen serving daily. The number of servings you need per day appears in parentheses.

Month ____________ **Week** __________

	S	M	T	W	TH	F	S
Daily weight (optional)							
Protein foods (4)							
Vitamin C foods (2)							
Calcium foods (4)							
Green leafy/Yellows (3 or more)							
Other fruits & vegetables (2 or more)							
Grains/Carbs. (5 or more)							
Iron-rich foods (some daily)							
Fat (2½-7½)							
Salt							
Fluids (8-10)							
Nutritional supplement							

Month ____________ **Week** __________

	S	M	T	W	TH	F	S
Daily weight (optional)							
Protein foods (4)							
Vitamin C foods (2)							
Calcium foods (4)							
Green leafy/Yellows (3 or more)							
Other fruits & vegetables (2 or more)							
Grains/Carbs. (5 or more)							
Iron-rich foods (some daily)							
Fat (2½-7½)							
Salt							
Fluids (8-10)							
Nutritional supplement							

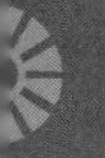

Your Daily Dozen Diary

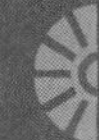

Check off each Daily Dozen serving daily. The number of servings you need per day appears in parentheses.

Month ___________ **Week** _________

	S	M	T	W	TH	F	S
Daily weight (optional)							
Protein foods (4)							
Vitamin C foods (2)							
Calcium foods (4)							
Green leafy/Yellows (3 or more)							
Other fruits & vegetables (2 or more)							
Grains/Carbs. (5 or more)							
Iron-rich foods (some daily)							
Fat (2½-7½)							
Salt							
Fluids (8-10)							
Nutritional supplement							

Month ___________ **Week** _________

	S	M	T	W	TH	F	S
Daily weight (optional)							
Protein foods (4)							
Vitamin C foods (2)							
Calcium foods (4)							
Green leafy/Yellows (3 or more)							
Other fruits & vegetables (2 or more)							
Grains/Carbs. (5 or more)							
Iron-rich foods (some daily)							
Fat (2½-7½)							
Salt							
Fluids (8-10)							
Nutritional supplement							

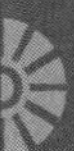

Your Daily Dozen Diary

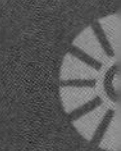

Check off each Daily Dozen serving daily. The number of servings you need per day appears in parentheses.

Month ___________ **Week** _________

	S	M	T	W	TH	F	S
Daily weight (optional)							
Protein foods (4)							
Vitamin C foods (2)							
Calcium foods (4)							
Green leafy/Yellows (3 or more)							
Other fruits & vegetables (2 or more)							
Grains/Carbs. (5 or more)							
Iron-rich foods (some daily)							
Fat (2½-7½)							
Salt							
Fluids (8-10)							
Nutritional supplement							

Month ___________ **Week** _________

	S	M	T	W	TH	F	S
Daily weight (optional)							
Protein foods (4)							
Vitamin C foods (2)							
Calcium foods (4)							
Green leafy/Yellows (3 or more)							
Other fruits & vegetables (2 or more)							
Grains/Carbs. (5 or more)							
Iron-rich foods (some daily)							
Fat (2½-7½)							
Salt							
Fluids (8-10)							
Nutritional supplement							

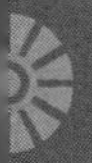

Your Daily Dozen Diary

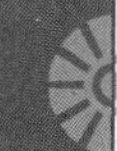

Check off each Daily Dozen serving daily. The number of servings you need per day appears in parentheses.

Month __________ **Week** ________

	S	M	T	W	TH	F	S
Daily weight (optional)							
Protein foods (4)							
Vitamin C foods (2)							
Calcium foods (4)							
Green leafy/Yellows (3 or more)							
Other fruits & vegetables (2 or more)							
Grains/Carbs. (5 or more)							
Iron-rich foods (some daily)							
Fat (2½-7½)							
Salt							
Fluids (8-10)							
Nutritional supplement							

Month __________ **Week** ________

	S	M	T	W	TH	F	S
Daily weight (optional)							
Protein foods (4)							
Vitamin C foods (2)							
Calcium foods (4)							
Green leafy/Yellows (3 or more)							
Other fruits & vegetables (2 or more)							
Grains/Carbs. (5 or more)							
Iron-rich foods (some daily)							
Fat (2½-7½)							
Salt							
Fluids (8-10)							
Nutritional supplement							

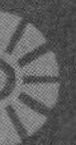

Your Daily Dozen Diary

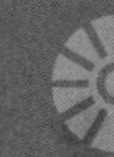

Check off each Daily Dozen serving daily. The number of servings you need per day appears in parentheses.

Month ___________ **Week** _________

	S	M	T	W	TH	F	S
Daily weight (optional)							
Protein foods (4)							
Vitamin C foods (2)							
Calcium foods (4)							
Green leafy/Yellows (3 or more)							
Other fruits & vegetables (2 or more)							
Grains/Carbs. (5 or more)							
Iron-rich foods (some daily)							
Fat (2½-7½)							
Salt							
Fluids (8-10)							
Nutritional supplement							

Month ___________ **Week** _________

	S	M	T	W	TH	F	S
Daily weight (optional)							
Protein foods (4)							
Vitamin C foods (2)							
Calcium foods (4)							
Green leafy/Yellows (3 or more)							
Other fruits & vegetables (2 or more)							
Grains/Carbs. (5 or more)							
Iron-rich foods (some daily)							
Fat (2½-7½)							
Salt							
Fluids (8-10)							
Nutritional supplement							

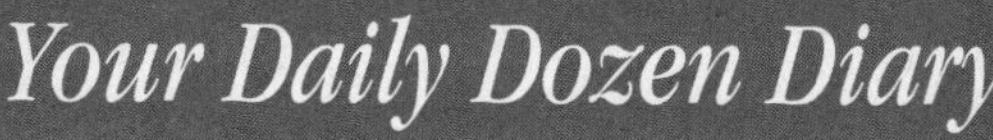
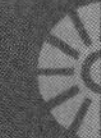

Your Daily Dozen Diary

Check off each Daily Dozen serving daily. The number of servings you need per day appears in parentheses.

Month ____________ **Week** __________

	S	M	T	W	TH	F	S
Daily weight (optional)							
Protein foods (4)							
Vitamin C foods (2)							
Calcium foods (4)							
Green leafy/Yellows (3 or more)							
Other fruits & vegetables (2 or more)							
Grains/Carbs. (5 or more)							
Iron-rich foods (some daily)							
Fat (2½-7½)							
Salt							
Fluids (8-10)							
Nutritional supplement							

Month ____________ **Week** __________

	S	M	T	W	TH	F	S
Daily weight (optional)							
Protein foods (4)							
Vitamin C foods (2)							
Calcium foods (4)							
Green leafy/Yellows (3 or more)							
Other fruits & vegetables (2 or more)							
Grains/Carbs. (5 or more)							
Iron-rich foods (some daily)							
Fat (2½-7½)							
Salt							
Fluids (8-10)							
Nutritional supplement							

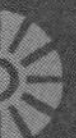

Your Daily Dozen Diary

Check off each Daily Dozen serving daily. The number of servings you need per day appears in parentheses.

Month ____________**Week** __________

	S	M	T	W	TH	F	S
Daily weight (optional)							
Protein foods (4)							
Vitamin C foods (2)							
Calcium foods (4)							
Green leafy/Yellows (3 or more)							
Other fruits & vegetables (2 or more)							
Grains/Carbs. (5 or more)							
Iron-rich foods (some daily)							
Fat (2½-7½)							
Salt							
Fluids (8-10)							
Nutritional supplement							

Month ____________**Week** __________

	S	M	T	W	TH	F	S
Daily weight (optional)							
Protein foods (4)							
Vitamin C foods (2)							
Calcium foods (4)							
Green leafy/Yellows (3 or more)							
Other fruits & vegetables (2 or more)							
Grains/Carbs. (5 or more)							
Iron-rich foods (some daily)							
Fat (2½-7½)							
Salt							
Fluids (8-10)							
Nutritional supplement							

Your Daily Dozen Diary

Check off each Daily Dozen serving daily. The number of servings you need per day appears in parentheses.

Month ___________ **Week** _________

	S	M	T	W	TH	F	S
Daily weight (optional)							
Protein foods (4)							
Vitamin C foods (2)							
Calcium foods (4)							
Green leafy/Yellows (3 or more)							
Other fruits & vegetables (2 or more)							
Grains/Carbs. (5 or more)							
Iron-rich foods (some daily)							
Fat (2½-7½)							
Salt							
Fluids (8-10)							
Nutritional supplement							

Month ___________ **Week** _________

	S	M	T	W	TH	F	S
Daily weight (optional)							
Protein foods (4)							
Vitamin C foods (2)							
Calcium foods (4)							
Green leafy/Yellows (3 or more)							
Other fruits & vegetables (2 or more)							
Grains/Carbs. (5 or more)							
Iron-rich foods (some daily)							
Fat (2½-7½)							
Salt							
Fluids (8-10)							
Nutritional supplement							

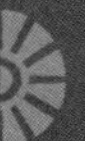

Your Daily Dozen Diary

Check off each Daily Dozen serving daily. The number of servings you need per day appears in parentheses.

Month ___________ **Week** _________

	S	M	T	W	TH	F	S
Daily weight (optional)							
Protein foods (4)							
Vitamin C foods (2)							
Calcium foods (4)							
Green leafy/Yellows (3 or more)							
Other fruits & vegetables (2 or more)							
Grains/Carbs. (5 or more)							
Iron-rich foods (some daily)							
Fat (2½-7½)							
Salt							
Fluids (8-10)							
Nutritional supplement							

Month ___________ **Week** _________

	S	M	T	W	TH	F	S
Daily weight (optional)							
Protein foods (4)							
Vitamin C foods (2)							
Calcium foods (4)							
Green leafy/Yellows (3 or more)							
Other fruits & vegetables (2 or more)							
Grains/Carbs. (5 or more)							
Iron-rich foods (some daily)							
Fat (2½-7½)							
Salt							
Fluids (8-10)							
Nutritional supplement							

Your Daily Dozen Diary

Check off each Daily Dozen serving daily. The number of servings you need per day appears in parentheses.

Month ___________ **Week** _________

	S	M	T	W	TH	F	S
Daily weight (optional)							
Protein foods (4)							
Vitamin C foods (2)							
Calcium foods (4)							
Green leafy/Yellows (3 or more)							
Other fruits & vegetables (2 or more)							
Grains/Carbs. (5 or more)							
Iron-rich foods (some daily)							
Fat (2½-7½)							
Salt							
Fluids (8-10)							
Nutritional supplement							

Month ___________ **Week** _________

	S	M	T	W	TH	F	S
Daily weight (optional)							
Protein foods (4)							
Vitamin C foods (2)							
Calcium foods (4)							
Green leafy/Yellows (3 or more)							
Other fruits & vegetables (2 or more)							
Grains/Carbs. (5 or more)							
Iron-rich foods (some daily)							
Fat (2½-7½)							
Salt							
Fluids (8-10)							
Nutritional supplement							

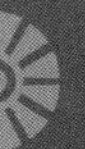

Your Daily Dozen Diary

Check off each Daily Dozen serving daily. The number of servings you need per day appears in parentheses.

Month ____________ **Week** __________

	S	M	T	W	TH	F	S
Daily weight (optional)							
Protein foods (4)							
Vitamin C foods (2)							
Calcium foods (4)							
Green leafy/Yellows (3 or more)							
Other fruits & vegetables (2 or more)							
Grains/Carbs. (5 or more)							
Iron-rich foods (some daily)							
Fat (2½-7½)							
Salt							
Fluids (8-10)							
Nutritional supplement							

Month ____________ **Week** __________

	S	M	T	W	TH	F	S
Daily weight (optional)							
Protein foods (4)							
Vitamin C foods (2)							
Calcium foods (4)							
Green leafy/Yellows (3 or more)							
Other fruits & vegetables (2 or more)							
Grains/Carbs. (5 or more)							
Iron-rich foods (some daily)							
Fat (2½-7½)							
Salt							
Fluids (8-10)							
Nutritional supplement							

Your Daily Dozen Diary

Check off each Daily Dozen serving daily. The number of servings you need per day appears in parentheses.

Month ___________ **Week** _________

	S	M	T	W	TH	F	S
Daily weight (optional)							
Protein foods (4)							
Vitamin C foods (2)							
Calcium foods (4)							
Green leafy/Yellows (3 or more)							
Other fruits & vegetables (2 or more)							
Grains/Carbs. (5 or more)							
Iron-rich foods (some daily)							
Fat (2½-7½)							
Salt							
Fluids (8-10)							
Nutritional supplement							

Month ___________ **Week** _________

	S	M	T	W	TH	F	S
Daily weight (optional)							
Protein foods (4)							
Vitamin C foods (2)							
Calcium foods (4)							
Green leafy/Yellows (3 or more)							
Other fruits & vegetables (2 or more)							
Grains/Carbs. (5 or more)							
Iron-rich foods (some daily)							
Fat (2½-7½)							
Salt							
Fluids (8-10)							
Nutritional supplement							

Your Daily Dozen Diary

Check off each Daily Dozen serving daily. The number of servings you need per day appears in parentheses.

Month ___________**Week** _________

	S	M	T	W	TH	F	S
Daily weight (optional)							
Protein foods (4)							
Vitamin C foods (2)							
Calcium foods (4)							
Green leafy/Yellows (3 or more)							
Other fruits & vegetables (2 or more)							
Grains/Carbs. (5 or more)							
Iron-rich foods (some daily)							
Fat (2½-7½)							
Salt							
Fluids (8-10)							
Nutritional supplement							

Month ___________**Week** _________

	S	M	T	W	TH	F	S
Daily weight (optional)							
Protein foods (4)							
Vitamin C foods (2)							
Calcium foods (4)							
Green leafy/Yellows (3 or more)							
Other fruits & vegetables (2 or more)							
Grains/Carbs. (5 or more)							
Iron-rich foods (some daily)							
Fat (2½-7½)							
Salt							
Fluids (8-10)							
Nutritional supplement							

Your Daily Dozen Diary

Check off each Daily Dozen serving daily. The number of servings you need per day appears in parentheses.

Month ____________ **Week** __________

	S	M	T	W	TH	F	S
Daily weight (optional)							
Protein foods (4)							
Vitamin C foods (2)							
Calcium foods (4)							
Green leafy/Yellows (3 or more)							
Other fruits & vegetables (2 or more)							
Grains/Carbs. (5 or more)							
Iron-rich foods (some daily)							
Fat (2½-7½)							
Salt							
Fluids (8-10)							
Nutritional supplement							

Month ____________ **Week** __________

	S	M	T	W	TH	F	S
Daily weight (optional)							
Protein foods (4)							
Vitamin C foods (2)							
Calcium foods (4)							
Green leafy/Yellows (3 or more)							
Other fruits & vegetables (2 or more)							
Grains/Carbs. (5 or more)							
Iron-rich foods (some daily)							
Fat (2½-7½)							
Salt							
Fluids (8-10)							
Nutritional supplement							

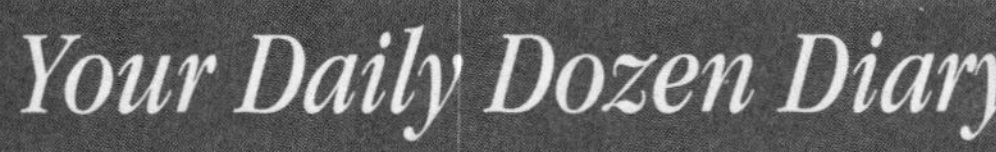

Your Daily Dozen Diary

Check off each Daily Dozen serving daily. The number of servings you need per day appears in parentheses.

Month ____________ **Week** __________

	S	M	T	W	TH	F	S
Daily weight (optional)							
Protein foods (4)							
Vitamin C foods (2)							
Calcium foods (4)							
Green leafy/Yellows (3 or more)							
Other fruits & vegetables (2 or more)							
Grains/Carbs. (5 or more)							
Iron-rich foods (some daily)							
Fat (2½-7½)							
Salt							
Fluids (8-10)							
Nutritional supplement							

Month ____________ **Week** __________

	S	M	T	W	TH	F	S
Daily weight (optional)							
Protein foods (4)							
Vitamin C foods (2)							
Calcium foods (4)							
Green leafy/Yellows (3 or more)							
Other fruits & vegetables (2 or more)							
Grains/Carbs. (5 or more)							
Iron-rich foods (some daily)							
Fat (2½-7½)							
Salt							
Fluids (8-10)							
Nutritional supplement							

Your Daily Dozen Diary

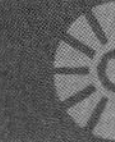

Check off each Daily Dozen serving daily. The number of servings you need per day appears in parentheses.

Month ____________ **Week** __________

	S	M	T	W	TH	F	S
Daily weight (optional)							
Protein foods (4)							
Vitamin C foods (2)							
Calcium foods (4)							
Green leafy/Yellows (3 or more)							
Other fruits & vegetables (2 or more)							
Grains/Carbs. (5 or more)							
Iron-rich foods (some daily)							
Fat (2½-7½)							
Salt							
Fluids (8-10)							
Nutritional supplement							

Month ____________ **Week** __________

	S	M	T	W	TH	F	S
Daily weight (optional)							
Protein foods (4)							
Vitamin C foods (2)							
Calcium foods (4)							
Green leafy/Yellows (3 or more)							
Other fruits & vegetables (2 or more)							
Grains/Carbs. (5 or more)							
Iron-rich foods (some daily)							
Fat (2½-7½)							
Salt							
Fluids (8-10)							
Nutritional supplement							

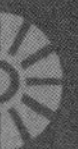

Your Daily Dozen Diary

Check off each Daily Dozen serving daily. The number of servings you need per day appears in parentheses.

Month ___________ **Week** _________

	S	M	T	W	TH	F	S
Daily weight (optional)							
Protein foods (4)							
Vitamin C foods (2)							
Calcium foods (4)							
Green leafy/Yellows (3 or more)							
Other fruits & vegetables (2 or more)							
Grains/Carbs. (5 or more)							
Iron-rich foods (some daily)							
Fat (2½-7½)							
Salt							
Fluids (8-10)							
Nutritional supplement							

Month ___________ **Week** _________

	S	M	T	W	TH	F	S
Daily weight (optional)							
Protein foods (4)							
Vitamin C foods (2)							
Calcium foods (4)							
Green leafy/Yellows (3 or more)							
Other fruits & vegetables (2 or more)							
Grains/Carbs. (5 or more)							
Iron-rich foods (some daily)							
Fat (2½-7½)							
Salt							
Fluids (8-10)							
Nutritional supplement							

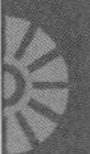

Your Daily Dozen Diary

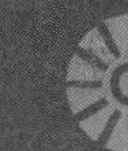

Check off each Daily Dozen serving daily. The number of servings you need per day appears in parentheses.

Month ____________ **Week** __________

	S	M	T	W	TH	F	S
Daily weight (optional)							
Protein foods (4)							
Vitamin C foods (2)							
Calcium foods (4)							
Green leafy/Yellows (3 or more)							
Other fruits & vegetables (2 or more)							
Grains/Carbs. (5 or more)							
Iron-rich foods (some daily)							
Fat (2½-7½)							
Salt							
Fluids (8-10)							
Nutritional supplement							

Month ____________ **Week** __________

	S	M	T	W	TH	F	S
Daily weight (optional)							
Protein foods (4)							
Vitamin C foods (2)							
Calcium foods (4)							
Green leafy/Yellows (3 or more)							
Other fruits & vegetables (2 or more)							
Grains/Carbs. (5 or more)							
Iron-rich foods (some daily)							
Fat (2½-7½)							
Salt							
Fluids (8-10)							
Nutritional supplement							

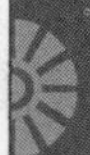

Your Daily Dozen Diary

Check off each Daily Dozen serving daily. The number of servings you need per day appears in parentheses.

Month ____________ **Week** __________

	S	M	T	W	TH	F	S
Daily weight (optional)							
Protein foods (4)							
Vitamin C foods (2)							
Calcium foods (4)							
Green leafy/Yellows (3 or more)							
Other fruits & vegetables (2 or more)							
Grains/Carbs. (5 or more)							
Iron-rich foods (some daily)							
Fat (2½-7½)							
Salt							
Fluids (8-10)							
Nutritional supplement							

Month ____________ **Week** __________

	S	M	T	W	TH	F	S
Daily weight (optional)							
Protein foods (4)							
Vitamin C foods (2)							
Calcium foods (4)							
Green leafy/Yellows (3 or more)							
Other fruits & vegetables (2 or more)							
Grains/Carbs. (5 or more)							
Iron-rich foods (some daily)							
Fat (2½-7½)							
Salt							
Fluids (8-10)							
Nutritional supplement							

Your Daily Dozen Diary

Check off each Daily Dozen serving daily. The number of servings you need per day appears in parentheses.

Month ____________ **Week** __________

	S	M	T	W	TH	F	S
Daily weight (optional)							
Protein foods (4)							
Vitamin C foods (2)							
Calcium foods (4)							
Green leafy/Yellows (3 or more)							
Other fruits & vegetables (2 or more)							
Grains/Carbs. (5 or more)							
Iron-rich foods (some daily)							
Fat (2½-7½)							
Salt							
Fluids (8-10)							
Nutritional supplement							

Month ____________ **Week** __________

	S	M	T	W	TH	F	S
Daily weight (optional)							
Protein foods (4)							
Vitamin C foods (2)							
Calcium foods (4)							
Green leafy/Yellows (3 or more)							
Other fruits & vegetables (2 or more)							
Grains/Carbs. (5 or more)							
Iron-rich foods (some daily)							
Fat (2½-7½)							
Salt							
Fluids (8-10)							
Nutritional supplement							

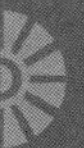

Your Daily Dozen Diary

Check off each Daily Dozen serving daily. The number of servings you need per day appears in parentheses.

Month ____________ **Week** __________

	S	M	T	W	TH	F	S
Daily weight (optional)							
Protein foods (4)							
Vitamin C foods (2)							
Calcium foods (4)							
Green leafy/Yellows (3 or more)							
Other fruits & vegetables (2 or more)							
Grains/Carbs. (5 or more)							
Iron-rich foods (some daily)							
Fat (2½-7½)							
Salt							
Fluids (8-10)							
Nutritional supplement							

Month ____________ **Week** __________

	S	M	T	W	TH	F	S
Daily weight (optional)							
Protein foods (4)							
Vitamin C foods (2)							
Calcium foods (4)							
Green leafy/Yellows (3 or more)							
Other fruits & vegetables (2 or more)							
Grains/Carbs. (5 or more)							
Iron-rich foods (some daily)							
Fat (2½-7½)							
Salt							
Fluids (8-10)							
Nutritional supplement							

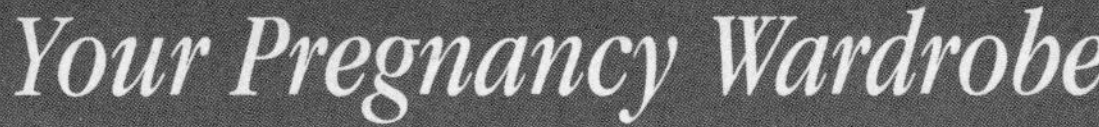

Your Pregnancy Wardrobe

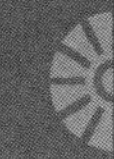

List what you can use from previous pregnancies, what's usable from your prepregnancy wardrobe, what you can borrow, and what you need to buy. Keep in mind that oversized shirts, sweatshirts, and T's (your own or your partner's) can serve admirably throughout your pregnancy and later as well.

Item	Source

Your Pregnancy Wardrobe

Item	Source

Notes

Notes

Getting Ready for Baby

3

Getting Ready for Baby

Between shopping for your own pregnancy wardrobe, a layette for baby, and a host of other necessities for your new life-with-baby, the local shopping center could easily become a second home. Use of this section can help you take stock of hand-me-downs, gifts, and purchases, making shopping trips more efficient—and possibly less frequent.

The Comparison Shopping pages will help you find the best buys on baby furnishings, from cribs to high chairs.

Of course, getting ready for baby means more than shopping. Use the Interview pages to assist you in selecting the best doctor to take care of your new arrival, and if you plan on hiring help, a baby nurse for the short haul or a nanny for the long.

Choosing a name you, your partner, and your baby can live with for the rest of all of your lives can be a monumental challenge. Meet it by using the Baby Name pages in this section.

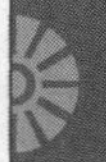

Baby Essentials

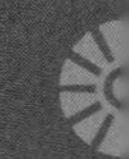

What You Will Need For Baby

The following list is a general guide for putting together baby essentials. Individualize it, depending on where you live, the time of year your baby will arrive, your lifestyle, and your budget. Take inventory of hand-me-downs as well as of gifts. Check off what you already have before heading for the stores. As you make purchases or place orders, check these off, too. Buy the larger quantities of each item if you do laundry once a week, the smaller if you do it more often.

But don't buy too much too soon. Infants don't stay tiny for very long and a sudden downpour of gifts at a baby shower could leave you with more than your baby could ever use. Keep in mind, too, that there will be more gifts once your baby arrives. To avoid duplicates, share this list with friends when they ask what you can use (or register at a baby store). And save receipts from your own purchases to make exchanges and returns easier.

THE LAYETTE

Item	Have	Need	Source
Diapers (one or a combination of the following):			
Diaper service			
4 dozen cloth diapers			
6 dozen disposables, newborn size (about 1 week's supply)			
1 dozen extra cloth diapers for miscellaneous uses			
3-6 waterproof pants, diaper covers, or diaper wraps (to use with cloth diapers)			
Diaper liners, for cloth diapers (optional)			

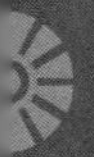

Baby Essentials

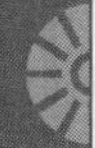

THE LAYETTE

Item	Have	Need	Source
3-7 undershirts			
2-3 blanket sleepers or 3-7 heavy weight sleepers (for fall or winter babies)			
3-7 lightweight sleepers (for spring or summer babies)			
2-4 pair booties or socks (all one color and style for easier pairing)			
3-7 stretch suits (seasonally appropriate)			
1-3 sweaters (seasonally appropriate)			
1 bunting or snowsuit bag with attached mitts (for fall or winter baby)			
Lightweight, brimmed hat (summer)			
Warm knit hat (winter)			
2-6 crib sheets			
1-2 waterproof mattress pads			
2-6 bassinet sheets (if applicable)			
1-2 crib-size blankets			
4-8 receiving blankets			
2-4 hooded bath towels			
2-4 baby washcloths			
2-4 washable bibs			

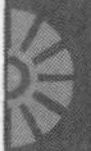

Baby Essentials

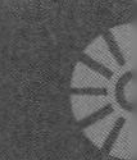

BABY TOILETRIES

Item	Have	Need	Source
Baby soap (bar or bath liquid)			
No-tears baby shampoo (or use baby soap instead)			
Baby cornstarch			
Ointment for diaper rash (ask practitioner for recommendation)			
Petroleum jelly			
Diaper wipes (alcohol-free)			
Sterile cotton balls			
8 diaper pins (if needed, for cloth diapers)			
Baby nail scissors or clippers			
Baby brush and comb			
Other			

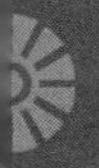

Baby Essentials

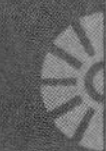

BABY'S MEDICINE CHEST

Get recommendations for specific items from the practitioner you've chosen.

Item	Have	Need	Source
Liquid acetaminophen			
Liquified charcoal (if recommended by local poison center)			
Syrup of Ipecac			
Saline nose drops			
Antiseptic cream			
Hydrogen peroxide			
Oral rehydration fluid			
Rubbing alcohol			
Calibrated medicine spoon, dropper, and/or oral syringe			
Sterile Band-Aids and gauze pads			
Adhesive tape			
Tweezers			
Infant nasal aspirator			
Vaporizer/humidifier			
Thermometer (standard rectal or tympanic)			
Small penlight			
Tongue depressors			
Heating pad and/or hot-water bottle			
Other			

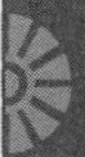

Baby Essentials

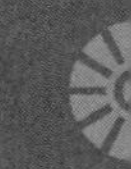

FEEDING SUPPLIES

Item	Have	Need	Source
If you're breastfeeding exclusively:			
1 baby bottle with nipple (for water or emergency supplement)			
Breast pump, if needed			
If you're bottle feeding exclusively or partially:			
4 bottles (4 ounces each) and 10-12 bottles (8 ounces each), with newborn nipple units			
Utensils for formula preparation			
Sterilizer, if recommended by your baby's practitioner			
Two-week supply of formula, as recommended by the practitioner			
Other			

FURNISHINGS*

Item	Have	Need	Source
Crib			
Crib mattress			
Bumpers			
Bassinet or cradle (optional)			
Changing table, pad, or space			
Diaper pail (if home laundering)			
Chest of drawers			
Baby bath tub			
Infant seat			
Other			

Baby Essentials

FOR BABY'S OUTINGS*

Item	Have	Need	Source
Car seat			
Baby carrier (optional)			
Diaper bag			
Stroller (optional)			
Carriage (optional)			
Combination stroller-carriage (optional)			
Portable crib (optional)			

OTHER

*For tips on safe buying, see *What to Expect the First Year.*

Comparison Shopping

Item

Store/Salesperson Phone

Make/Style

Size Color Price

Delivery/Availability

Features

Item

Store/Salesperson Phone

Make/Style

Size Color Price

Delivery/Availability

Features

Item

Store/Salesperson Phone

Make/Style

Size Color Price

Delivery/Availability

Features

Comparison Shopping

Item

Store/Salesperson Phone

Make/Style

Size Color Price

Delivery/Availability

Features

Item

Store/Salesperson Phone

Make/Style

Size Color Price

Delivery/Availability

Features

Item

Store/Salesperson Phone

Make/Style

Size Color Price

Delivery/Availability

Features

Comparison Shopping

Item

Store/Salesperson Phone

Make/Style

Size Color Price

Delivery/Availability

Features

Item

Store/Salesperson Phone

Make/Style

Size Color Price

Delivery/Availability

Features

Item

Store/Salesperson Phone

Make/Style

Size Color Price

Delivery/Availability

Features

Comparison Shopping

Item

Store/Salesperson Phone

Make/Style

Size Color Price

Delivery/Availability

Features

Item

Store/Salesperson Phone

Make/Style

Size Color Price

Delivery/Availability

Features

Item

Store/Salesperson Phone

Make/Style

Size Color Price

Delivery/Availability

Features

Comparison Shopping

Item

Store/Salesperson Phone

Make/Style

Size Color Price

Delivery/Availability

Features

Item

Store/Salesperson Phone

Make/Style

Size Color Price

Delivery/Availability

Features

Item

Store/Salesperson Phone

Make/Style

Size Color Price

Delivery/Availability

Features

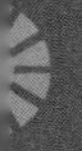

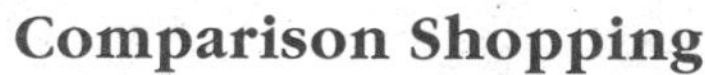

Comparison Shopping

Item

Store/Salesperson Phone

Make/Style

Size Color Price

Delivery/Availability

Features

Item

Store/Salesperson Phone

Make/Style

Size Color Price

Delivery/Availability

Features

Item

Store/Salesperson Phone

Make/Style

Size Color Price

Delivery/Availability

Features

Comparison Shopping

Item

Store/Salesperson Phone

Make/Style

Size Color Price

Delivery/Availability

Features

Item

Store/Salesperson Phone

Make/Style

Size Color Price

Delivery/Availability

Features

Item

Store/Salesperson Phone

Make/Style

Size Color Price

Delivery/Availability

Features

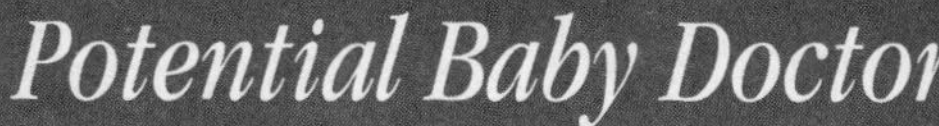

Potential Baby Doctor

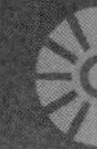

Interview Notes

Name

Address

Phone

Specialty, training

Hospital affiliation

Office hours Typical waiting time

Call hours

House call policy

Office smoking policy

Type of practice (solo, group, HMO, etc.)

If group, will you always see same doctor?

Will you have a choice?

Is a nurse-practitioner part of practice?

How much well-baby care does he/she provide?

Who fills in when doctor isn't available?

What protocol is followed in emergencies?

What protocol is followed with sick children (eg: separate office hours)?

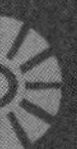

Potential Baby Doctor

Doctor's attitude toward issues you care about:

breastfeeding

preventative medicine

circumcision

nutrition

vegetarianism

antibiotic use

other

Your observations:

waiting room environment

examination room environment

staff/doctor attitude toward children

staff/doctor attitude toward parents

your comfort with doctor

Notes

Potential Baby Doctor

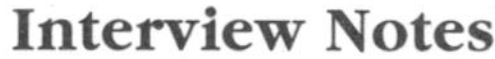

Interview Notes

Name

Address

Phone

Specialty, training

Hospital affiliation

Office hours — Typical waiting time

Call hours

House call policy

Office smoking policy

Type of practice (solo, group, HMO, etc.)

If group, will you always see same doctor?

Will you have a choice?

Is a nurse-practitioner part of practice?

How much well-baby care does he/she provide?

Who fills in when doctor isn't available?

What protocol is followed in emergencies?

What protocol is followed with sick children (eg: separate office hours)?

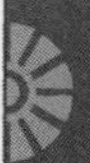

Potential Baby Doctor

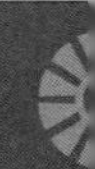

Doctor's attitude toward issues you care about:

breastfeeding

preventative medicine

circumcision

nutrition

vegetarianism

antibiotic use

other

Your observations:

waiting room environment

staff

staff/doctor attitude toward children

staff/doctor attitude toward parents

your comfort with doctor

Notes

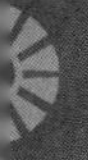

Potential Baby Doctor

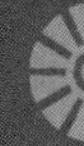

Interview Notes

Name

Address

Phone

Specialty, training

Hospital affiliation

Office hours Typical waiting time

Call hours

House call policy

Office smoking policy

Type of practice (solo, group, HMO, etc.)

If group, will you always see same doctor?

Will you have a choice?

Is a nurse-practitioner part of practice?

How much well-baby care does he/she provide?

Who fills in when doctor isn't available?

What protocol is followed in emergencies?

What protocol is followed with sick children (eg: separate office hours)?

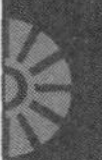

Potential Baby Doctor

Doctor's attitude toward issues you care about:

breastfeeding

preventative medicine

circumcision

nutrition

vegetarianism

antibiotic use

other

Your observations:

waiting room environment

staff

staff/doctor attitude toward children

staff/doctor attitude toward parents

your comfort with doctor

Notes

Potential Baby Doctor

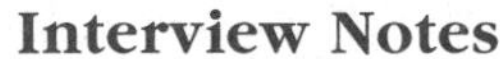

Interview Notes

Name ______________________________

Address ______________________________

Phone ______________________________

Specialty, training ______________________________

____

Hospital affiliation ______________________________

Office hours ______________ Typical waiting time ______________

Call hours ______________________________

House call policy ______________________________

Office smoking policy ______________________________

Type of practice (solo, group, HMO, etc.) ______________________________

If group, will you always see same doctor? ______________________________

Will you have a choice? ______________________________

Is a nurse-practitioner part of practice? ______________________________

How much well-baby care does he/she provide? ______________________________

____

Who fills in when doctor isn't available? ______________________________

What protocol is followed in emergencies? ______________________________

____

What protocol is followed with sick children (eg: separate office hours)? ______________________________

____

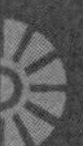

Potential Baby Doctor

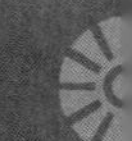

Doctor's attitude toward issues you care about:

breastfeeding

preventative medicine

circumcision

nutrition

vegetarianism

antibiotic use

other

Your observations:

waiting room environment

staff

staff/doctor attitude toward children

staff/doctor attitude toward parents

your comfort with doctor

Notes

Potential Baby Nurse

Interview Notes

Name

Address Phone

Recommended by

Agency, if any

Appointment date Time

Training and/or experience

Fee Date available Hours available

Sleep in/out

Attitude toward breastfeeding

Willingness to include both parents in babycare

Willingness to teach you the ropes

Willingness to do: Cooking Light cleaning

Laundry Heavy cleaning

Willingness to care for older siblings

Health and TB status

References (be sure to check them)

1.

2.

3.

Notes

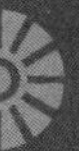

Potential Baby Nurse

Interview Notes

Name

Address | Phone

Recommended by

Agency, if any

Appointment date | Time

Training and/or experience

Fee | Date available | Hours available

Sleep in/out

Attitude toward breastfeeding

Willingness to include both parents in babycare

Willingness to teach you the ropes

Willingness to do: Cooking | Light cleaning

Laundry | Heavy cleaning

Willingness to care for older siblings

Health and TB status

References (be sure to check them)

1.

2.

3.

Notes

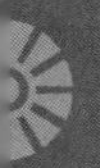

Potential Baby Nurse

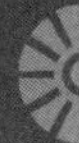

Interview Notes

Name ______________________________

Address ______________________ Phone ______________

Recommended by ______________________________

Agency, if any ______________________________

Appointment date ______________________ Time ______________

Training and/or experience ______________________________

Fee ______________ Date available ______________ Hours available ______________

Sleep in/out ______________________________

Attitude toward breastfeeding ______________________________

Willingness to include both parents in babycare ______________________________

Willingness to teach you the ropes ______________________________

Willingness to do: Cooking ______________ Light cleaning ______________

Laundry ______________ Heavy cleaning ______________

Willingness to care for older siblings ______________________________

Health and TB status ______________________________

References (be sure to check them) ______________________________

1. ______________________________

2. ______________________________

3. ______________________________

Notes ______________________________

____

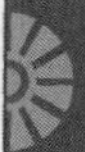

Potential Baby Nurse

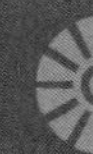

Interview Notes

Name

Address Phone

Recommended by

Agency, if any

Appointment date Time

Training and/or experience

Fee Date available Hours available

Sleep in/out

Attitude toward breastfeeding

Willingness to include both parents in babycare

Willingness to teach you the ropes

Willingness to do: Cooking Light cleaning

Laundry Heavy cleaning

Willingness to care for older siblings

Health and TB status

References (be sure to check them)

1.

2.

3.

Notes

Potential Baby Nurse

Interview Notes

Name

Address | Phone

Recommended by

Agency, if any

Appointment date | Time

Training and/or experience

Fee | Date available | Hours available

Sleep in/out

Attitude toward breastfeeding

Willingness to include both parents in babycare

Willingness to teach you the ropes

Willingness to do: Cooking | Light cleaning

Laundry | Heavy cleaning

Willingness to care for older siblings

Health and TB status

References (be sure to check them)

1.

2.

3.

Notes

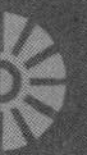

Selecting a Name for Baby

For many expectant parents, few tasks are as challenging as choosing a name for the new baby. Sometimes listing the candidates, along with their meanings and the reasons for considering them, makes it easier to evaluate and compare them. Use these pages for that purpose in the months prior to delivery…and may the best name win!

Names Under Consideration

First	Middle	Meaning/Derivation	Source/Namesake

Selecting a Name for Baby

First	Middle	Meaning/Derivation	Source/Namesake

Selecting a Name for Baby

First	Middle	Meaning/Derivation	Source/Namesake

Your Baby Shower

Date

Place

Hosted by

Memorable moments

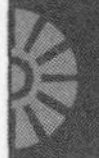

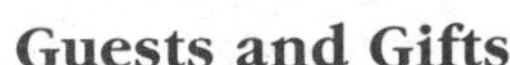

Guests and Gifts

Guest	Gift	Thank-You Sent

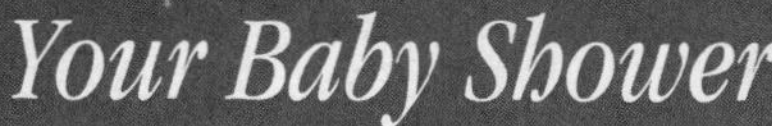

Guests and Gifts

Guest	Gift	Thank-You Sent

Notes

Getting Ready for Childbirth

4

Getting Ready for Childbirth

Childbirth doesn't usually last much longer than 24 hours, and is sometimes over in three or four. Yet preparation for this momentous event takes a good deal more time. To make sure you're ready when baby is, begin your preparations early. Use this section to take childbirth class notes, to develop a birthing plan to discuss with your practitioner, to itemize what you'll need to pack for the hospital, to list people to call when you go into labor or after you deliver, and people to whom you want to send announcements.

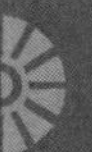

Childbirth Education Class

Date Time

Place Teacher

Class Notes

Homework

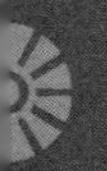

Childbirth Education Class

Date Time

Place Teacher

Class Notes

Homework

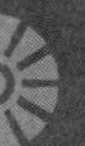

Childbirth Education Class

Date Time

Place Teacher

Class Notes

Homework

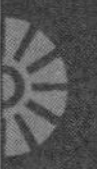

Childbirth Education Class

Date

Time

Place

Teacher

Class Notes

Homework

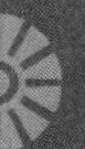

Childbirth Education Class

Date Time

Place Teacher

Class Notes

Homework

Childbirth Education Class

Date Time

Place Teacher

Class Notes

Homework

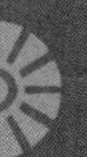

Childbirth Education Class

Date

Time

Place

Teacher

Class Notes

Homework

Childbirth Education Class

Date Time

Place Teacher

Class Notes

Homework

Birthing Plan

To minimize miscommunications and misunderstandings later, put any concerns and preferences you may have about labor and delivery down on paper now. Discuss your wishes with your practitioner well in advance of your due date. Your birthing plan should include any of the following that are important to you.*

Going to hospital earlier (or later) in labor than is usual

Eating and/or drinking during labor

Walking about, sitting up, staying in bed during labor

Wearing contact lenses during labor and delivery (usually not permitted if general anesthesia used)

Locale of labor and delivery—birthing room, labor room, delivery room

*For a discussion of each of these issues, see *What to Expect When You're Expecting*. Remember that, because of physician judgment or hospital policy, some of these may not be negotiable. Even when all parties have agreed to a birthing plan in advance, an unexpected turn of events at delivery may require changes.

Birthing Plan

Personalizing labor environment with music, lighting, items from home

Use of a still camera or video camera during labor and/or delivery

Administration of an enema

Shaving of the pubic area

Routine starting of an intravenous line for administration of fluids, pain medication, or labor-stimulating drugs

Use of pain medication

Routine catheterization (to drain urine from the bladder)

Fetal monitoring (continuous, intermittent, portable); internal (scalp) fetal monitoring

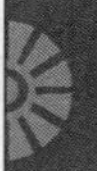

Birthing Plan

Induction of labor or augmentation of contractions with oxytocin

Delivery positions (squatting, semi-sitting, supine, etc.)

Routine episiotomy; use of massage or other techniques to reduce need for episiotomy

Forceps/vacuum cap use

Cesarean section; VBAC (vaginal birth after previous cesarean)

Nasal suctioning of the newborn; suctioning by the father, partner, or labor coach

Timing of cutting the umbilical cord; who cuts the cord

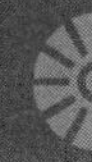

Birthing Plan

Presence of significant others (in addition to your spouse, partner, coach, or doula) during labor and/or delivery

Presence of older children at or immediately after delivery

Holding the baby immediately after birth; breastfeeding immediately after birth

Postponing weighing baby and administering eye drops until after you and your baby have met

Your presence at weighing of baby, administration of eye drops, first pediatric exam, and baby's first bath

Baby's feeding schedule while in hospital (will it be governed by nursery's schedule or your baby's hunger?)

Birthing Plan

Availability of support for breastfeeding in the hospital

Management of breast engorgement if you're not planning to breastfeed

Circumcision

Rooming in for baby and for other parent

Hospital visitation for children/other relatives

Postpartum medication and procedures

Length of the hospital stay with uncomplicated vaginal delivery; with a cesarean section

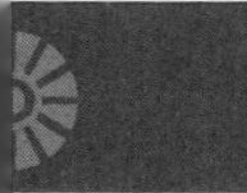

Birthing Plan

Other

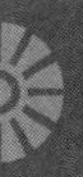

Hospital Checklist

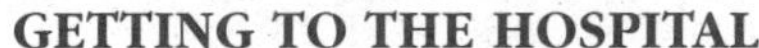

GETTING TO THE HOSPITAL

Jot down the following well in advance of your due date.

Cab company name/phone no.	
Friend or relative who can drive you/phone no.	
Best route	
Parking garages open 24 hours, if needed	
Hospital entrance to use	
Department to report to	
Ambulance service/phone no.	

PACKING FOR THE LABOR OR BIRTHING ROOM

Have these packed and ready in advance of your due date, too.

Cash for cab fare	
Plenty of change for telephone calls and snack machines	
Health insurance card and forms, if applicable	
Camera/film; video or audio recorder/cassettes (if you're planning to photograph or tape the event)	
Watch or clock with second hand for timing contractions	

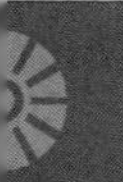

Hospital Checklist

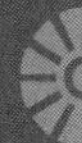

Lotion for massages	
Small paper bag to treat hyperventilation	
Tennis ball or rolling pin for countermassage during back labor	
Sugarless lollipops or sucking candies to keep your mouth moist	
Heavy socks for cold feet	
Split of Champagne or sparkling cider labeled with your name (for celebrating)	
Toss in at the last minute: *The Pregnancy Organizer, What to Expect When You're Expecting, What to Expect the First Year*	

PACKING FOR YOUR HOSPITAL ROOM

Hospitals often provide personal care products, but feel free to bring your own favorites. Keep in mind your hospital stay may be no more than 24 hours.

Robe/bed jacket	
Nightgown	
Slippers	
Perfume, non-talc powder, cosmetics, toothbrush, toothpaste	
Soap, deodorant, skin lotion, shampoo, conditioner	
Hair brush, hair dryer, curling iron	
Playing cards, books or magazines, writing paper, other distractions	
Packs of raisins, nuts, whole-grain crackers, and nutritious snacks	
List of names to call (see Who to Call After Delivery)	

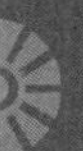

Going Home Checklist

Have these packed and ready before you give birth and either take them along or have them brought in on the day before you leave the hospital (keep in mind that you may stay for only 24 hours).

FOR MOM	
A roomy (you won't be back to prepregnancy shape) outfit to go home in	
Bra (nursing bra if you plan to breastfeed)	
Panties	
Slip, if needed	
Shoes	
Hosiery	
Coat or sweater, if necessary	
Tote or shopping bag for gifts and hospital supplies	
Other	

FOR BABY	
T-shirt	
Kimono or stretch suit	
Booties	
Receiving blanket	
Sweater in cool weather	
Knitted hat in cool weather	
Bunting or blanket in cold weather	
2 disposable diapers (though hospital will probably provide some)	
Infant car seat	
Other	

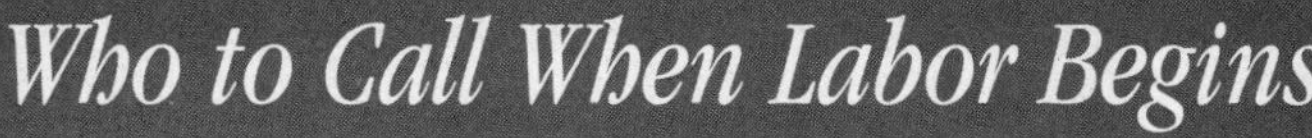
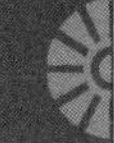

Who to Call When Labor Begins

Names and Numbers

Spouse/Partner

Practitioner

Coach

Doula

Hospital

Parents (yours and your spouse's)

Siblings (yours and your spouse's)

Baby-sitter for other children

Neighbors/Friends/Co-workers

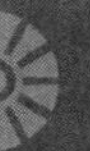

Who to Call After Delivery

Names and Numbers

Childbirth educator

Diaper service (if using)

Insurance company

Baby nurse (if using)

Store deliveries (layette, crib,other furnishings, etc.)

Stationer to order announcements

Other family members/Friends/Co-workers

Notes

Notes

Baby's Arrival

5

Baby's Arrival

With the contractions coming strong and fast, you may think that labor is an experience you'll never forget. But chances are, as soon as it's over, the details will quickly begin to fade. Exactly when did those first contractions start? When did you leave for the hospital? How long did you push? What, if any, medication, did you have? In order to be able to reliably relay this information to your practitioners during future pregnancies, to pass this bit of family lore on to your children and grandchildren, and to reminisce about it yourself, jot down the particulars as they happen (or delegate the job to someone else) in the pages that follow. Also record the first moments you share with your baby, what he or she looks like, his or her Apgar scores, and other vital statistics.

In the Postpartum pages, you can record how your baby's first feedings progress, how you feel physically and emotionally, and important early milestones. Also record instructions from the pediatrician, your own practitioner, and the hospital or nursery nurses on the designated pages.

Use the album pages to mount a baby announcement and the planning pages to organize a baby naming, baptism, christening, ritual circumcision, or any other baby-related celebration.

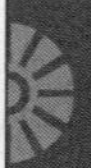

Labor Diary

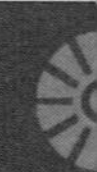

Date and time contractions first began

How far apart were they? How long did each last?

What did they feel like?

Where were you?

What were you doing?

Who was with you?

When had you last eaten and what did you have?

How did you react?

How did you contact your spouse/partner, if you were not together?

How did your spouse/partner react?

Labor Diary

How did your older children, if any, react?

When did you call your practitioner?

What instructions were you given?

How did you pass the time at home?

When did you go to the hospital?

How did you get there?

With whom?

If this was a false alarm, use the following note pages for subsequent starts. If labor has started, continue recording contractions periodically in the Contraction Record.

Notes

Notes

Labor Diary

Contraction Record

Time Starts	Duration	Time Starts	Duration

Time now

How far apart are contractions now (from start to start)?

How long does each last (from start to finish)?

Time Starts	Duration	Time Starts	Duration

Time now

How far apart are contractions now (from start to start)?

How long does each last (from start to finish)?

Labor Diary

Contraction Record

Time Starts	Duration	Time Starts	Duration

Time now

How far apart are contractions now (from start to start)?

How long does each last (from start to finish)?

Time Starts	Duration	Time Starts	Duration

Time now

How far apart are contractions now (from start to start)?

How long does each last (from start to finish)?

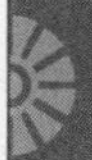

Labor Diary

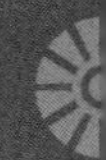

Contraction Record

Time Starts	Duration	Time Starts	Duration

Time now

How far apart are contractions now (from start to start)?

How long does each last (from start to finish)?

Time Starts	Duration	Time Starts	Duration

Time now

How far apart are contractions now (from start to start)?

How long does each last (from start to finish)?

Labor Diary

Contraction Record

Time Starts	Duration	Time Starts	Duration

Time now

How far apart are contractions now (from start to start)?

How long does each last (from start to finish)?

Time Starts	Duration	Time Starts	Duration

Time now

How far apart are contractions now (from start to start)?

How long does each last (from start to finish)?

Contraction Record

Time Starts	Duration	Time Starts	Duration

Time now

How far apart are contractions now (from start to start)?

How long does each last (from start to finish)?

Time Starts	Duration	Time Starts	Duration

Time now

How far apart are contractions now (from start to start)?

How long does each last (from start to finish)?

Contraction Record

Time Starts	Duration	Time Starts	Duration

Time now

How far apart are contractions now (from start to start)?

How long does each last (from start to finish)?

Time Starts	Duration	Time Starts	Duration

Time now

How far apart are contractions now (from start to start)?

How long does each last (from start to finish)?

Labor Diary

Contraction Record

Time Starts	Duration	Time Starts	Duration

Time now

How far apart are contractions now (from start to start)?

How long does each last (from start to finish)?

Time Starts	Duration	Time Starts	Duration

Time now

How far apart are contractions now (from start to start)?

How long does each last (from start to finish)?

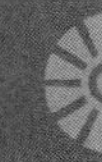

Labor Diary

Contraction Record

Time Starts	Duration	Time Starts	Duration

Time now

How far apart are contractions now (from start to start)?

How long does each last (from start to finish)?

Time Starts	Duration	Time Starts	Duration

Time now

How far apart are contractions now (from start to start)?

How long does each last (from start to finish)?

First Stage: Labor

First (early or latent) phase of labor (contractions 5–20 minutes apart; cervix 0–3 cm. dilatation)

Began

Comments

Second (active) phase of labor (contractions 3–4 minutes apart; cervix 3–7 cm. dilated)

Began

Comments

Third (active or transitional) phase of labor (contractions 2–3 minutes apart, 60–90 seconds long; cervix 7–10 cm. dilated)

Began

Comments

Anesthesia or medication during labor, if any

Induction or augmentation of labor, if any

Comments

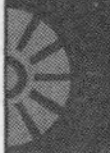

Second Stage: Delivery

Vaginal Delivery

Where you delivered

Birth attendants

You began pushing at | Delivery position

Anesthesia or medication (and reaction), if any

Type of episiotomy, if any

Complications, if any

Baby born at | Placenta delivered at

Comments

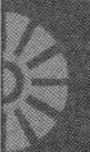

Surgical Delivery

Reason for

Birth attendants

Type of anesthesia (and reaction), if any

Baby born at | Placenta delivered at

Comments

Notes

Notes

Notes

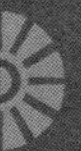

Meet the Baby

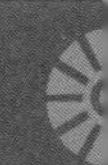

Vital Statistics

Weight ______ Length ______

Head circumference ______ Chest circumference ______

Test Results

Apgar at 1 minute ______ Apgar at 5 minutes ______

Brazelton test ______

PKU test ______

Other tests ______

Other procedures ______

Results of First Physical Exam

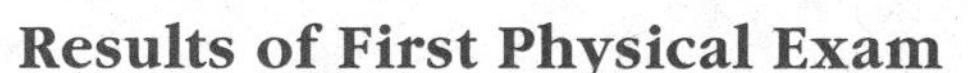

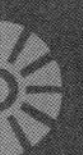

Meet the Baby

Appearance

Hair

Eyes

Birthmarks

Looks like

Has mother's

Has father's

Other features/characteristics

Baby's Name

First

Middle

Named for

Nickname, if any

Birth certificate filed

Date Social Security no. applied for

First Photo

(attach here)

Reactions

First meeting with Mommy

First meeting with Daddy

Meet the Baby

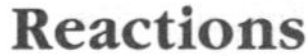

Reactions

First meeting with sibling(s)

First meeting with grandparents/other family members

First Feeding Experiences

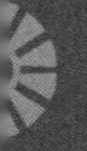

Baby Care Instructions

Note instructions from nurses or doctor.

Feeding

Bathing

Cord care

Baby Care Instructions

Care of circumcision, if applicable

Other instructions

When to call for baby's first well-baby visit

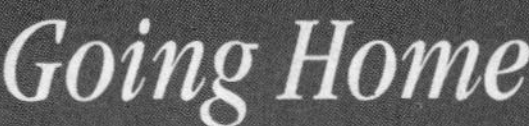

Going Home

Discharged from the hospital on

Traveled home via

Who was with you?

How did you feel?

What did you do when you first arrived home?

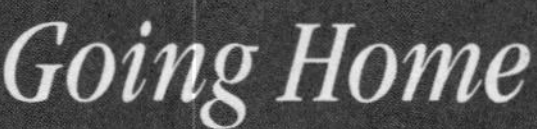

Going Home Photo

attach here

Birth Announcements

Name	Address	Sent

Birth Announcements

Name	Address	Sent

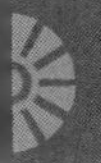

Birth Announcements

Name	Address	Sent

Birth Announcements

Name	Address	Sent

Your Baby's Birth Announcement

(attach here)

Baby Gifts

Gift	From	Thank-You Sent

Baby Gifts

Gift	From	Thank-You Sent

Baby Gifts

Gift	From	Thank-You Sent

Baby Gifts

Gift	From	Thank-You Sent

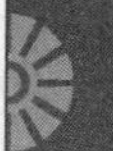

Special Events and Celebrations

Event

Date

Menu

Guest list

Celebration Diary

Special Events and Celebrations

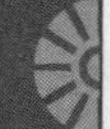

Event

Date

Menu

Guest list

Celebration Diary

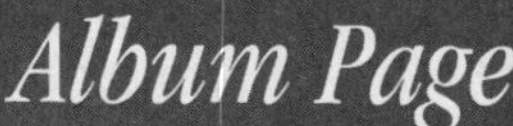

Album Page

Baby's Photo

(attach here)

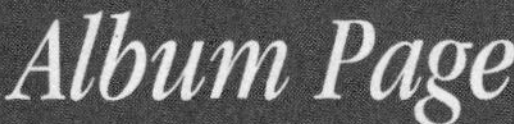

Album Page

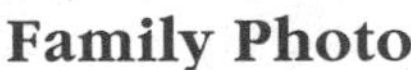

Family Photo

(attach here)

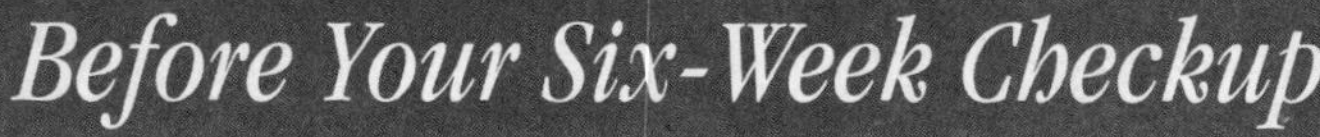

Before Your Six-Week Checkup

Calls Made to Practitioner

Date Called

Reason

Practitioner's response/instructions

Date called

Reason

Practitioner's response/instructions

Questions to Ask at the Next Visit

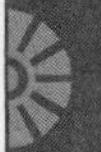

Your Six-Week Checkup

Appointment Date

Practitioner

Date Time

Your weight

Your blood pressure

Other tests

PAP smear

Method of birth control selected, if any

Prescription number, if any

Diaphragm size, if any

Next appointment

Practitioner's Instructions

Notes

Notes

Notes